OSTEOPOROSIS CURE AND TREATMENT HANDBOOK

AN ULTIMATE GUIDE TO HEALING OF OSTEOPOROSIS

DR HALEA WORKMAN

Table of Contents

CHAPTER ONE

Treatment of osteoporosis

Because osteoporosis weakens bones, they are more easily broken by stress or trauma. Bone fractures are often the only sign that the disease has progressed and is no longer dormant. Preventative measures and treatments are available if you want to avoid contracting this disease.

Osteoporosis is a term that refers to a variety of conditions.

Osteoporosis, or "porous bone," is the medical term for this condition. Bone fractures are more likely if you have this disease, which weakens bones and puts you at risk for them. Osteoporosis is a condition in which bone mass and strength are reduced over time. In many cases, the disease goes undetected until a bone fracture is painful and necessitates a lengthy hospital stay. Hip, wrist, and spine fractures are the most common.

Osteoporosis can affect anyone.

Osteoporosis affects an estimated 200 million people worldwide. About 54 million people live in the United States. Both sexes can develop osteoporosis, but women are four times more likely to suffer from it than men. Two million men in the United States currently suffer from osteoporosis, and another 12 million are at risk of developing the disease.

After the age of 50, one in two women and one in four men will suffer an osteoporotic fracture. Another 30 percent of the population is at risk of developing osteoporosis because of their low bone density. Osteopenia is the medical term for this condition.

There are more than two million fractures each year due to osteoporosis, and this number is only going up. Osteoporosis can be prevented if you take certain precautions. Osteoporosis can also be slowed by treatment, but it's not a cure.

Osteoporosis can be explained even if researchers don't know why it occurs. Bones are made of living tissue, and they grow and change. Bones that are in good health look like sponges on the inside. Trabecular bone is the term for this area. The spongy bone is surrounded by a hard outer shell. Cortical bone refers to the outer layer of bone.

"Holes" form in the "sponge," weakening the inside of the bone, as osteoporosis progresses. Bones provide structural support and provide vital organs with protection. Calcium and other minerals can also be found in bones. Bone is broken down and rebuilt when the body needs calcium. Bone remodeling is a process that provides the body with the calcium it needs while also preserving the strength of the bones.

Until the age of 30 or so, you're more likely to build bone than you are to lose it. There is a gradual decrease in bone mass after the age of 35 because the breakdown of bone occurs faster than the growth of bone. Osteoporosis causes you to lose bone mass more quickly. In postmenopausal women, bone loss accelerates even more rapidly.

Osteoporosis is characterized by what?

Osteoporosis usually has no symptoms. As a result, the

disease is sometimes called "silent." There are, however, some things to be aware of:

• A decrease in height (getting shorter by an inch or more).

• Adjustment of body position (stooping or bending forward).

A feeling of being out of breath (smaller lung capacity due to compressed disks).

Fractures of the skeleton.

• Lower back pain.

Osteoporosis can affect anyone.

Gender and age are two of the most significant risk factors for developing osteoporosis, but there are many others.

Osteoporosis fractures become more common as people get older. Osteoporosis is most common in women over the age of 50 or those who have gone through menopause. In the first decade following menopause, women experience rapid bone loss because estrogen production, a hormone that protects against excessive bone loss, slows.

CHAPTER TWO

Osteoporosis and aging affect both men and women. Men over the age of 50 are more likely than younger men to suffer an osteoporosis-induced bone fracture. In the United States, about 80,000 men are expected to break a hip each year, and men are more likely to die in the year following a hip fracture.

Osteoporosis risk is also influenced by your ethnicity. Osteoporosis is more common in Caucasian and Asian women than in any other ethnic group.

African-American and Hispanic women, on the other hand, remain at risk. African-American women, on the other hand, are more likely than white women to die following a hip fracture.

It's also important to consider bone structure and body weight as additional variables. Osteoporosis is more likely to strike petite and thin people because they have less bone mass to compensate for bone loss.

Having a history of osteoporosis in one's family can also increase one's chances of developing the disease. You may be at greater risk of developing osteoporosis if your parents or grandparents have shown any signs of the disease, such as a fractured hip following a minor fall.

Finally, certain medical conditions and medications can put you at greater risk of harm. Earlier screening for osteoporosis may be recommended if you or your healthcare provider have or have had any of the following conditions, some of which are linked to irregular hormone levels.

• Thyroid, parathyroid, or adrenal glands that are overactive.

• Weight loss surgery or organ transplantation history.

A history of missed periods or a diagnosis of breast or prostate cancer necessitates hormone therapy.

Asthma or Crohn's disease. • Celiac disease.

Multiple myeloma is one example of a blood disease.

Osteoporosis can occur as a side effect of some medications. Steroids, breast cancer treatments, and seizure medications are among these. Talk to your doctor or pharmacist about how your medications affect your bones.

Every risk factor may appear to be linked to something beyond your control, but this isn't the case. Some of the risk factors for osteoporosis are under your control. If you have questions or concerns about your medication, talk to your doctor or nurse practitioner. And you're in charge of your:

Osteoporosis is more likely to occur if you don't get enough calcium and vitamin D in your diet. Although bulimia and anorexia are risk factors, treatment is possible.

• Sedentary (inactive) lifestyles are associated with a higher risk of osteoporosis.

Fractures are more likely to occur in people who smoke.

Osteoporosis is more likely to occur if you drink at least two drinks a day.

PHYSIOLOGY AND LAB TESTS

How do you know if you have osteoporosis?

Before any problems arise, your doctor or other medical professional can order a bone density test for you. A DXA scan or a DEXA scan are other names for bone mineral density (BMD) tests. Radiation from these X-rays is used to determine the strength of your spine, hip, or wrist bones. Osteoporosis can only be detected by regular X-rays when the disease is advanced.

Bone density tests should be performed on all women over 65. For women who have risk factors for osteoporosis, the DEXA scan may be done earlier. Men over the age of 70, as well as younger men with certain risk factors, should think about getting their bone density checked.

The treatment of osteoporosis

Exercise, vitamin and mineral supplements, and medications are all options for those with already-diagnosed osteoporosis. Osteoporosis prevention often involves a combination of exercise and dietary supplementation. All three types of exercise—weight bearing, resistance, and balance—are critical.

Osteoporosis medications fall into a variety of categories. Your healthcare provider will work with you to find the best solution. For osteoporosis, there isn't really a single best medication. The treatment that is best for you is the one that is best for you.

Treatments involving hormones

Raloxifene is a selective estrogen receptor modulator, and it is included in this class.

Among women who are experiencing menopausal symptoms or who are younger than menopause, estrogen therapy is more common because of the risk of blood clots, cancer, and heart disease that goes along with it.

If your testosterone levels are low, your doctor may prescribe testosterone to help you build stronger bones.

To the bones, raloxifene has an estrogenic effect. Taken every day, the medication comes in tablet form. Raloxifene may also be used to reduce the risk of breast cancer in some women, in addition to treating osteoporosis. Five years of raloxifene treatment is generally recommended for the treatment of osteoporosis.

In the form of Fortical® and Miacalcin®, calcitonin-salmon is a man-made hormone. A reduction in spine fractures but not hip fractures or other types of fractures can be achieved by using this product It can either be injected or inhaled through the nose, depending on the patient's preference. For the inhaled form, side effects may include a runny nose or nosebleed as well as headaches. For the injected form, side effects include rashes and flushing. It's not a good idea to use it as your first option. More serious side effects, such as a possible link to cancer, are also possible.

Bisphosphonates

Treatments with bisphosphonate phosphates for osteoporosis are antiresorptive. They prevent the body from reabsorbing bone tissue. You can choose from a variety of dosage schedules (monthly, weekly, and even yearly), as well as different brands of medication.

These include Fosamax, Fosamax Plus D , and Binosto

Boniva is the brand name for ibandronate.

• Actonel and Atelvia are the two most commonly prescribed risedronate drugs.

• Zoledronic acid: Reclast

After three to five years of taking bisphosphonates, you may be able to stop and still receive benefits. There are also generic versions of these medicines. Boniva and Atelvia are only suitable for women, while the others can be used by both genders.

Bisphosphonates may cause flu-like symptoms (fever, headache), heartburn, and decreased kidney function, among other side effects. Osteonecrosis of the jaw or atypical femur fractures are rare but serious side effects that should be considered (low trauma fractures of the thigh). Long-term (>5-year) use of the medication increases the risk of these uncommon side effects.

Biologics

Denosumab is an injection that can be given to both men and women every six months. When other treatments have failed, it is frequently used as an alternative. This medication can be used even in cases where kidney function has declined. The long-term effects of this drug are unknown, but there are possible side effects that could be life-threatening. Bones in the thigh or jaw may be fractured or infected, as well as serious infection.

steroid hormones

Osteoporosis sufferers can benefit from the use of these products. There are currently three of these products on the market:.

For postmenopausal women who are at a high risk of fracture, the FDA has approved Evenity. Both new bone formation and decreased bone breakdown are facilitated by the product. Once a month, you'll receive two injections, one right after the other. These injections have a one-year expiration date.

During the course of two years, patients receive daily injections of teriparatide (Forteo) and abaloparatide (Tymlos). In many ways, they are parathyroid hormones, or products that resemble the hormones in many ways.

CHAPTER THREE

When is it appropriate to use medication to treat osteoporosis?

The risk of fracture in women with a T score of -2.5 or lower, like -3.3 or -3.8, should be addressed with therapy right away. Osteopenia, a milder form of bone thinning than osteoporosis, necessitates medical attention for many women. Your doctor may use the WHO fracture risk assessment tool (FRAX) to determine if you need treatment based on your risk factors and bone density results. Osteoporosis fractures, such as those of the wrist, spine, or hip, should also be addressed by medical professionals (sometimes even if the bone density results are normal).

Supplements

Despite the fact that dietary supplements are widely available over-the-counter and online, they are not subject to the same level of regulation as prescription medications. This should be kept in mind. Even if a substance is referred to as "natural," it does not necessarily mean that it is safe for everyone to consume at any given time.

You may be advised by your doctor to eat a diet rich in calcium and vitamin D. If you have osteoporosis or are trying to prevent it, this is critical. Ideally, you should be able to meet those needs through a food plan, but that may not be possible. A number of algae-based calcium supplements are on the market.

Diet and/or supplementation with 1,000-1,200 mg of calcium

per day is recommended. A higher intake of calcium has not been shown to increase bone strength, but it may increase the risk of kidney stones, calcium buildup in blood vessels, and constipation.

Vitamin D levels vary widely, but it is true that many people do not have adequate levels and may need to take supplements. Your doctor may conduct a blood test and then make a recommendation based on the results of that test.

Osteoporosis has been linked to a number of other supplements. One of these is strontium, which has never been approved in the United States for the treatment of osteoporosis.. Strontium ranelate, a prescription drug in the European Union, has been taken off the market because of serious side effects.

The risks and benefits of taking a prescription drug or dietary supplement should always be discussed with your doctor.

Osteoporosis can be prevented in several ways.

Osteoporosis can be prevented by modifying your diet and lifestyle. Restoring estrogen levels with hormone therapy helps postmenopausal women avoid osteoporosis.

Diet

You need to eat a diet high in calcium to keep your bones strong and healthy throughout your life. Calcium is found in one cup of skim or 1% fat milk.

Salmon, sardines, kale, broccoli, calcium-fortified juices and breads, dried figs, and calcium supplements are all excellent calcium sources in addition to dairy products. Food and drink are the best sources of calcium.

As a supplement for those who need it, keep in mind that the body can only take in 500 mg of calcium at one go. Taking calcium supplements in large doses will not be absorbed, so you should take them in smaller doses.

THE END